Detox: 30 Cleansing Recipes For A Renewed You

A Drink A Day To Keep The Doctor Away, Boost Metabolism, Lose Weight, Look And Feel Great

Joseph J. Miller

© 2016

Disclaimer

This book is not intended as a substitute for the medical advice of physicians. The reader should regularly consult a physician in matters relating to his/her health and particularly with respect to any symptoms that may require diagnosis or medical attention.

Detox:

A Drink A Day To Keep the Doctor Away, Boost Metabolism, Lose Weight And Look Great

Chapter 1
What is a Detox?

When you hear the word detox, many things may come to mind. Detox is a hot topic today and has grabbed the attention of many health professionals as well as people looking to lose weight or just give their body the break it needs to function at the most optimal level.

A detox can be defined as a period of time where you are giving your body what it needs in order to rid itself of built up toxins, and clean the blood. A detox can also be described as a time for resting, cleaning, and nourishing the body from the inside out. (1) When you remove and eliminate toxins, and fuel your body with powerful nutrients the detox process can help you maintain overall health. Detoxification can be done for a number of reasons. Some people chose to detox seasonally in order to be sure they are getting their tune up in a few times a year. Other people may detox once per year or to try to kick start weight loss. Whatever the reason is behind detox, if done the proper way, detoxification can be extremely beneficial to one's overall health and wellbeing.

A detox works by helping your body to eliminate built up toxins. On an everyday basis, your kidneys, lungs, skin, intestines, and lymph system are responsible for excreting toxins but when these organs are not working at an optimal level, proper detox cannot take place. When you go on a detox you replenish your body and allow these organs to release the toxins and do the job they are meant to do.

Throughout this book I will discuss how a detox is beneficial, how a detox effects each individual organ, how to detox, and supply you with 30 detox recipes to get you started on your detox journey!

How is a Detox Beneficial?

A detox is beneficial for a number of reasons. Detoxification of the body can help to replenish the body and renew the organs while also cleaning your system. A detox can help the body's natural cleaning process through various different mechanisms.

Detox first and foremost allows the organs to rest, especially when you are on a fasting detox. Allowing organs such as the liver to rest is essential for allowing the liver to return to optimal functioning. When the liver is taxed and overburdened it will not work the way it should, and toxins will not be excreted. Detoxing will help to give each organ a rest, and allow the smooth removal of toxins.

A detox can also promote elimination from the intestines, skin, and the kidneys. When you are detoxing you want elimination to happen. Elimination is how toxins are going to be removed from the body. A detox can also benefit the blood and circulatory system in the body. Circulation can improve and the blood will be cleansed. A detox will ensure that you are refueling your body with the proper nutrients it needs. It's important to supply your body with extra nourishing foods during detoxification into order to support excretion and removal of toxic waste.

If you are someone who is looking to lose weight, starting on a detox is not only excellent for your overall health, it is also a great way to kick start weight loss. When you are abstaining from processed and artificial foods and only consuming nourishing juices and detoxifying smoothies, your ability to lose weight significantly increases. Allowing your organs the chance to let go of toxic waste can also assist with weight loss since toxins often get trapped in fat cells with can make trying to lose weight difficult.

Why Everyone Should Detox:

Almost everyone would benefit from going on a healthy and clean detox. Most people experience symptoms that signifies a detox is needed. Some of the reasons why someone should or needs to detox are if they experience constant unexplained fatigue, sluggish elimination, skin issues, allergies, dark circles or bags under the eyes, bloating, menstrual problems for women, and frequent mental confusion. All of these symptoms point towards toxin overload.

Everyone should detox at least once per year in order to cleanse the body. Many of the symptoms people may experience on an everyday basis will greatly improve after a detox. With the amount of pollution, artificial products, pesticides, chemicals and other harmful things we are exposed to everyday it's important to assist the body in removing those chemicals since our natural detoxification system is often times overloaded. Environmental toxins are linked to neurological diseases, cancer, stroke, heart disease and much more so making sure are bodies are able to detoxify these chemicals out is essential to maintaining health. (2)

Another reason why everyone should detox is to just restore balance to our bodies. When our bodies are so overloaded with toxins from foods, stress, and environmental toxins our body systems are not able to work together like they should. When our body systems are not working in unison it creates illness. Detoxing can help to bring the balance back to our internal systems and get us back on track.

Chapter 2: How Does a Detox Affect the Body?

In this section, I am going to discuss how detox affects multiple parts of the body.

Organ Function: Detoxing the body can greatly improve our organ function. As we have discussed, an overburdened body leaves us with built up toxins with the inability to actually excrete them. When it comes to detox, the point is to give all of our organs a break from the stress and work they do to keep our bodies running and allow them to rest and repair so they can refresh and work optimally again after detox. Some of the major organs that benefit the most include the liver, the intestines, and the kidneys. The liver benefits so much because when you are not consuming processed or toxic foods the liver does not have to work so hard in order to create these toxins into water soluble molecules and get them ready for excretion. The kidneys benefit in a similar way because they can take a break from having to be overworked by not having to excrete various toxins that are coming from liver detoxification. Both the liver and kidneys can have a break and start excreting the toxins that have been built up over days, months, or even years in a more natural way with the assistance of nourishing and detoxifying foods. The intestines also get a break because they also will not have to work so hard. Inflammation will reduce, and undigested foods can start to work their way out of your body. Improved digestion is a huge benefit that comes from a detox.

Digestive Function: After a detox you may notice a huge improvement with your digestion. A detox can help to boost the digestive system and help it to function properly. When your digestive system is working properly, your immune system also has the chance to function correctly since ¾ of your immune system is actually in your digestive tract. (3) When we are consuming inflammatory foods, our body can sometimes trigger an immune response, which can affect digestive health. When this occurs things like bloating, indigestion, acid reflux, and constipation can happen. Part of your immune system in your gut is also covered by a very thin lining that can easily be damaged by consuming processed, inflammatory foods. When this is damaged you are more susceptible to developing food allergies, and digestive conditions. "Your gut is also full of healthy bacteria that assists in breaking down and digesting food as well as serving as a first line of defense to eliminate toxins from your food." (4) An excess of chemicals, preservatives, and antibiotics can cause an imbalance in this bacteria can cause you to have a hard time digesting foods, regulating hormones, and excreting toxins. When your gut health is out of balance, dysbiosis can also developed, and imbalance in gut flora. When you are promoting healthy gut flora through a healthy detox, you are lowering the amount of energy needed to digest your food, which makes it harder for bad bacteria to cause disease. (4)

With a damaged digestive system, you may also be dealing with nutrient malabsorption. Since digestive health is a key player in the health of many other body functions, it is essential that it is working at its most optimal level. With the amount of toxins our bodies are exposed to on a daily basis, from the toxins we breathe in, to the toxins that we ingest there are countless digestive issues that can surface. A thorough detox can help to improve many of your gut issues, and leave your digestive system renewed and ready to work again. Think of it as a vacation for your gut, our gut also needs a little time to relax just like we do from time to time.

When we detox, the digestive system has a chance to absorb all of the nutrients coming in. If you are suffering with nutrient absorption issues, a detox will help to ensure that nutrients are getting in to the places they need to in order to heal your gut. That layer we talked about that is actually part of your immune system in your gut also has a chance to heal. When this repairs itself, digestion improves and so does your immune function. Inflammation will also reduce when things like gluten, dairy, sugar, caffeine and processed foods are removed from the diet. The gut can become inflamed when foods like grains, sugar, and dairy are consumed and the only way to cool that inflammation is by removing those foods and supporting your body with detoxifying foods instead. When the inflammation is reduce, acid reflux may improve, IBS symptoms may disappear, and things like constipation may no longer be an issue.

Weight Loss: Some people may start a detox in order to lose weight, and this is not necessarily a bad thing, but you have to do it the right way. When you begin a detox that is full of nourishing detoxifying foods such as fruit and vegetable smoothies and juices you will be on track to kick start weight loss. Some of the healthy ingredients in a detox drink that can help to flush out toxins and excess fat include cucumber, parsley, cilantro, and celery. Foods and herbs like this have healing properties that help your body let go of built up toxins. Many of the built up toxins eventually get stored as fat cells if they are not able to be excreted. Once the toxins are stored as fat, it takes a long time for them to be released and the only way to do so is when your body has the nourishment it requires for proper detox. If you are looking to lose weight, starting on a 3-5 day detox can help you get started on the right track. Take a look at the 3 day sample detox plan in chapter 4 for how to get started.

Immune System: Detoxification can play a huge role in improving your immune system. When our bodies are over stressed, out immune system like other organs is not able to work as efficiently as it should and you may be getting sick more than you should be. Your immune system improves with detox for a number of reasons. The first and most obvious reason is that your body is clearing out toxins. When these toxins are sitting in your body they have the ability to fire an immune response causing an inflammatory response, which could result in illness. The second reason why a detox helps to improve your immune system is during a detox or cleanse, you are avoiding thing like sugar and caffeine, which can both, suppress the immune system. Detoxing can also help to raise the pH in your body and make your body more alkaline. When you at more of an acidic state, you are much more likely to get sick. Alkaline foods such as fruits and vegetables are highly encouraged during a detox and the primary foods that will be consumed. An improved digestive system goes hand in hand with a strong immune system, and as we discussed a detox helps to repair a damaged immune system and help it function properly. In turn, the boosted digestive system will play a part in boosting your immune system as well. Doing a detox a few times a year can actually be more beneficial to your immune system than the pharmaceutical methods of boosting immune health.

Mental Health: It is not only the physical things that improve after doing a detox; it can also be how you feel mentally. It's all about aligning the body during detox, and improve our organ function. "When the body's systems are aligned, a shift also occurs with our mental and emotional states." (5) Once our body's system are aligned and balance we are able to take on more and handle more emotionally while also being able to make clearer decisions and see things in a more positive light. Foods that generally make you feel lethargic such as sugar, and processed foods are completed eliminated during a detox which allows clearer thinking and a reduction in "brain fog'

Stress: Part of detoxing the body also means incorporating some stress reduction self-care practices into your daily life. Stress can be a huge contributor to toxic overload on our bodies, so it's important to remove stress from our daily life. Some stress reducing recommendations to do during detox includes meditation, yoga, and walking. Moving our bodies and clearing our minds at the same time as cleaning our bodies is the best way to get the most out of a detox. If you practice stress reduction during a detox, you will see even better results in your overall health.

Chapter 3

How to Prepare for a Detox

Now that we have discussed all of the ways that a detox can be beneficial for your health, you may be ready to get started! Preparing for a detox doesn't have to be stressful; it can actually be even easier than your usual meal prep for the week. A liquid detox generally last for a minimum of 3 days but can last for up to 7. Going any longer than this may result in doing more harm than good. When you are preparing you want to keep in mind how many days you are choosing to detox in order to prepare everything that you need, so you stay on track. With anything in life success comes with preparation. You want to have a plan of action before you begin your detox and feel prepared before starting. I have created guidelines for you to follow to help get you started on your detox journey. Let's look at what you are going to need in order to prepare to detox your body.

How to Prepare:

This may sound funny, however the first thing you need to prepare for a detox is a positive attitude and understanding why you are starting this detox! Make sure to get really clear about your health goals and your "why" for doing this. If you have your health goals at the forefront of your mind throughout the detox you will most likely stick to it even when cravings set in. You may even want to make a list of your health goals and place in on your fridge for a friendly reminder.

The second thing you will need to do prior to detox, is adapting to a healthy lifestyle a few days before the cleanse. This is important, so that it's not a sudden shock and you will have an easier time staying on track throughout the detox. You will want to start replacing bad habits with healthier habits. For example, start swapping out your bag of chips with lunch everyday with some veggies with hummus, and start to reduce caffeine and completely eliminate soda. Some other things to avoid at least 3 days before a detox include animal products, all processed foods, including pastas, breads and salad dressings, alcohol, dairy, fried foods, eggs, and over salted foods. Try replacing these foods with things like beans, lentils, nuts and seeds, fruits, vegetables, salads, homemade soups and homemade salad dressings. Small changes a few days or a week before the detox will be incredibly beneficial, and will set the tone for long-term healthy changes. Another thing you can start to do is begin to incorporate just 5 minutes of meditation into your day, whenever you have time. This will help to kick start the stress reduction process. Starting a healthier lifestyle a little while before a cleanse can also help to prevent any cleansing symptoms, which can help make the detox go smoothly.

The final thing to do in terms of preparation is to remove all the processed foods from your pantry and refrigerator. If it is not there, you will not eat it. Removing it completely will also help to keep these foods out of your kitchen long term, and not just during the detox. Also be sure to let your loved ones know that you are doing a detox, and what your health goals are so that they can help to keep you on track. A strong support system is very helpful when trying to start your health journey.

Kitchen Supplies:

When detoxing, you will need a few kitchen supplies to make things easy. Below are my top choices of kitchen supplies for detox, as well as my top 10 detox ingredients for juices or smoothies.

Supplies:

- **High speed blender:** I like the Vitamix, because this can serve as a juicer as well. To use this blender as a juicer, simple blend up all of your ingredients, and strain into a large glass. You can also use a Nutribullet, or any other blender of your choice.

- **Re-usable glass containers:** These come in handy when you are making some juices or smoothies ahead of time. They can be used to store excess and placed in the fridge for later use. I prefer glass so that you are not being exposed to toxic reside that comes from plastic containers.

- **Juicer:** You can find juicers from as low as $50 up to over a thousand dollars. Whatever your choice is, a juicer is an excellent tool to have during and after your detox. If purchasing a juicer is not an option for you right now, do not worry you can use your blender and strain the smoothie to make it into a juice. Keep in mind that using the blender method will require more ingredients in order to make enough liquid for a juice.

- **Highly Quality Knife:** This will come in handy when it comes time to chop your veggies.

- **Re-usable Storage Bags:** Re-usable storage bags works great for storing chopped up fruits or veggies to make a grab and go smoothie or juice. Your detox should not be stressful, so having ingredients at your fingertips makes things easier and less stressful.

My top 10 Detox foods to have in Your Kitchen during a Detox:

- Cucumbers
- Celery
- Parsley
- Lemon
- Beets
- Ginger
- Turmeric
- Spinach
- Apples
- Kale

How Long Should You Detox For?

This is a question frequently asked before someone starts a detox. There are some time fame guidelines to follow in order to make sure you are detoxing the healthy way. Some detox programs recommend that you detox for almost an entire month. The problem with detoxing so long is that it will actually start to do more harm than good if you decide to detox for longer than a week. Detoxing for long periods of time can shut down your bowel function and actually prevent detoxification since your liver requires key nutrients in order to fully perform proper detoxification. These are 2 things you want the opposite of when starting a detox.

The recommended time frame for a safe detox is 3-7 days. A week or less is the perfect amount of time to allow your body to cleanse itself and start to repair organ function, since the body does require a little bit of time to really fully cleanse itself. Followed by a 3-7 day fruit and vegetable juice cleanse you should always follow that will a 5 day detox food plan to still allow your body to release toxins, while slowly introducing solid foods again. (6) Going from a juice fast right back into eating processed foods is going to erase all the hard work your body just did to cleanse itself, so it's important to stay on the healthy path and continue to follow a detoxification eating plan directly after a juice fast.

How Soon Will You See Benefits From A Detox?

When you decide to commit to a detox, you may be wondering how soon you will see benefits. With any cleanse the possibility of experiencing some cleansing symptoms such as digestive distress and headaches are always possible. Starting to eat cleaner and removing toxins such as tobacco and alcohol from your diet prior to detoxing is a good way to help to eliminate some of the cleansing symptoms. If you do experience cleansing symptoms, these will happen before you see a noticeable change in the way you feel on a detox. If you are experiencing some uncomfortable symptoms such as headache or stomach distress know that this will pass, and it is you bodies way of removing built up toxins. Stay positive and know that the feeling of health and wellbeing will come after the cleansing phase.

If you are deciding to detox for a whole 7 days you can expect to feel energized and renewed around day 3. After 3 whole days of allowing your body too flush out toxins that have been stagnant for a long period of time, the cleansing symptoms should be at bay, and you should be starting to see a change in how you feel. Around day 3 is also when those sugar cravings start to go away, which means you have made it over the hump! Keep going and you will feel even better once you hit day 7 of your week long detox.

How to Fight off Sugar Cravings during a Detox?

Sugar cravings are huge during a detox. It is naturally for us to crave something we have been so used to putting into our bodies. When we begin the detox process, we are removing all of the foods that are causing inflammation and toxin overload in our bodies, and cravings can definitely happen.

During the first 2 days of a detox is when the sugar cravings can really set in. You just started your cleanse, your body is in shock from not being fed all of the toxic foods, and it has begun the cleansing process. You may feel ill and all you want to do is crab something that is full of sugar that you think will make you feel better. Sugar is like a drug, and has actually been referred to as a drug because of how it acts in the body. Realize that this will pass, and once you resist the urge to feed your body with toxic sugar, you will find resisting it will become easier and easier. The detox process in not easy, especially the first couple of days however it does become easier, and by day 7 you will not even want sugar.

If you are experiencing an intense sugar craving one of the things you can do is make a juice will lots of lemon. Not only is lemon very cleansing, and alkalinizing it also can help to kick that sugar craving. You can also grab a large glass of water. A lot of time when we think that we are hungry, we are really just thirsty, but our minds are telling us to eat. Try to hydrate a little bit, and see if the craving goes away. Getting outside and removing yourself from your kitchen or any place where sugar cravings are triggered for you can be incredibly helpful. Get outside and take a brisk walk to eliminate the craving. Lastly, breathing is another trick to really help when these cravings occur. Take 5 cleansing deep breaths and take a look at your note you wrote about why you started this health journey. Sometimes all we need is a little reminder to keep us motivated and some cleansing breaths to calm the mind.

What To Do After A Detox?

After a detox, you want to stick to a healthy eating plan. For 5 straight days after a juice detox it is important to continue to eat detoxifying foods. 5 days after the detox, your body could still use a boost to continue the cleansing process, and fueling your body with detoxifying foods is the perfect way to continue to repair organ function. After a detox, it is important to start eating more raw foods. You can start by trying to eat 1 raw meal per day, which could consist of a nutritious fruit salad, a large salad for lunch or a refreshing green smoothie. Adding in 1 raw meal per day after a juice detox can help to continue to boost your energy levels, improve your skin, help you lose weight and even give you a more positive outlook on healthy eating. You can also add vegetables to every meal during the day. Try adding sautéed spinach to your pasture raised egg omelet in the morning, some chopped veggies in your salad at lunch and a side of steamed veggies for dinner. Getting your vegetables in everyday can be easy when you are mindfully adding them to every dish. Being sure to eat detoxifying foods throughout the day can be essential for continuing the cleansing process. Some great foods to eat include cruciferous vegetables such as broccoli, Brussel sprouts and cauliflower. Turmeric, ginger, garlic and onions are excellent additions to season any dish. Beets can be very cleansing and can be added to a smoothie, or a salad, and cucumber and celery can be great to cleanse the liver, and kidneys.

Continuing on your cleansing path after your juice detox can be essential for life long health changes. The detox is the kick-start, and what you do after is going to set the stage for how you should be taking care of your body lifelong.

Chapter 4

A 3-Day Sample Detox Diet Plan

Day 1	Day 2	Day 3
Breakfast Drink: Green Juice	Breakfast Drink: Green Juice	Breakfast Drink: Energizing Green Juice
Sample Supplement: Probiotic & high quality multi-vitamin	Sample Supplement: Probiotic & high quality multi-vitamin	Sample Supplement: Probiotic & high quality multi-vitamin
Lunch Drink: Coconut Milk Smoothie	Lunch Drink: Tropical Juice	Lunch Drink: Alkaline Juice
Snack: Repeat Green Juice	Snack: Repeat Green Juice	Snack: Repeat Energizing Green Juice
Dinner: Green Detox Juice	Dinner: Ginger Zing	Dinner: Heart Health Smoothie
Beverages: Water with lemon throughout the day	Beverages: Water with lemon throughout the day	Beverages: Water with lemon throughout the day

Recipes:

Please note that some of the recipes seen above are located in the recipe section in the last chapter of this book.

Green Juice

Ingredients: 6-8 leaves kale, 2 green apples, 1 cucumber, peeled, 2-3 stalks celery, 1/2 lemon (no peel), 2 inches fresh ginger, 1 cup water.

Coconut Milk Smoothie

Ingredients: 1 cup canned coconut milk, 1 frozen banana, 1 handful of fresh spinach, 1 handful of mint leaves. Blend until smooth.

Green Detox Juice

Ingredients: 2 celery stalks, chopped, 1 small cucumber, chopped, 2 kale leaves, 1 handful spinach, Handful of fresh parsley, 1 lemon peeled, 1 apple, seeded, cored and cut into chunks. Run all ingredients through a juicer, and enjoy.

30 Detox Recipes And The

Health Benefits Of Each

Tropical Juice

Ingredients:

- 1 stalk of celery
- 1 cucumber
- 2 cups of spinach leaves
- 1 cup of pineapple
- ½ cup of mango
- ½ lemon

Health Benefits:

- This smoothie is loaded with health benefits from each of the ingredients. The celery, and cucumber will help to flush out toxins and give the kidneys a boost, while the lemon will help to alkalinize the body. The pineapple is also high in papain, which is an enzyme that can be very beneficial to digestive health.

Ginger Zing

Ingredients:

- 1 stalk of celery
- 1 cucumber
- ½ inch of fresh ginger
- 1 handful of fresh parsley
- 1 lemon
- 1 apple
- 1 handful of fresh spinach

Health Benefits:

This ginger juice is full of anti-inflammatory properties that will help fight inflammation and nourish your body to return it to an alkaline state. The celery and cucumber will give this juice the ability to flush out toxins, while the ginger will fight inflammation, and the parsley will help to clean the blood. You may also notice that your breath is fresh after drinking this juice, which is another added benefit from the parsley.

Beet Juice

Ingredients:

- ¼ inch of fresh ginger
- 3 beets
- 3 stalks of celery
- 1 lemon

Health Benefits:

This juice is excellent for your liver, and digestive system. The beets will help to flush out toxins from the liver while also giving your digestive system a boost. The ginger will fight inflammation while the lemon will help to clean and alkalinize the blood.

Green Pear Juice

Ingredients:

- 1 handful of fresh spinach

- 1 pear

- 1 lemon

- 2 stalks of celery

- 1 cucumber

Health Benefits:

This refreshing juice will have your body detox in no time. The lemon and cucumber are very cleansing, and the spinach can help to fight cancer, and strengthen your body.

Anti-inflammatory Juice

Ingredients:

- ½ inch of fresh turmeric
- 4 carrots
- ¼ inch of fresh ginger
- 1 orange
- 1 lemon
- 2 stalks of celery

Health Benefits:

This is a powerhouse juice. If you are looking to fight off inflammation, this is the juice to grab. The turmeric and ginger act as anti-inflammatory agents in the body. Turmeric has been shown to work even better than NSAID medications to fight off pain and inflammation. The orange will help to give your immune system a boost, while the carrots can help to protect your vision as well as boost skin health.

Energizing Green Juice

Ingredients:

- 1 cucumber
- 1 handful of fresh cilantro
- 1 handful of fresh parsley
- 1 green apple
- 1 lemon
- ½ inch of fresh ginger
- 1 beet

Health Benefits:

If you are in need of an energy boost, try this energizing green juice. The tanginess from the apple, lemon and ginger will give you the perk up that you need while also helping to fight inflammation and reduce free radicals in your body. The cilantro will also help to detoxify your liver while parsley will help to clean the blood.

Avocado Smoothie (Blend)

Ingredients:

- 1 avocado, pitted, halves and skin removed
- 1 cup of canned coconut milk
- 1 handful of spinach
- 1 frozen banana
- 1 handful of ice

Health Benefits:

Raw spinach is very high in health benefits to help to rid of the body of toxins. Avocados can also help with detox and can help to reduce cholesterol levels. Coconut milk can help to provide you with energy, and is easy to digest. This is a great smoothie if you are looking for something a little more substantial than a juice.

Tropical Carrot Juice

Ingredients:

- 4 carrots
- ½ inch fresh ginger
- 1 green apple
- 1 lemon
- 1 cucumber
- 1 stalk of celery
- 1 handful of parsley

Health Benefits:

Carrots contain a unique property that assists in detox as well as hormone balance. The combination of ingredients in this juice work together to greatly detox the body. The celery will help to flush out toxins from the kidneys, as well as the cucumber, and the juice has overall ant inflammatory properties.

Alkaline Booster

Ingredients:

- 1 cucumber
- 2 stalks of celery
- 1 lemon
- 1 green apple
- 1 cup of leafy greens

Health Benefits:

This alkaline green juice has the ability to reduce acidity in the body and permeate it with alkalinizing foods. Since juices are so easily digested, your body will be able to take advantage of all of the alkaline benefits from each of these foods. The leafy greens will help to reduce acidity, while the cucumber, celery, lemon, and apple will help to remove built up toxins, and remove them from the body.

Sunshine Juice

Ingredients:

- 3 stalks of celery
- ½ cucumber
- 1 lemon
- 1 handful of parsley
- 1 green apple
- 1 cup kale

Health Benefits

This is a great juice to enjoy first thing in the morning, to give you a great kick-start. The tart flavors from the lemon, and green apple will help to boost your energy, while the kale can help rid your body of toxins through the liver. The parsley can also help to flush the kidneys of any build up salt, which can result in detoxification of other accumulated toxins as well.

Blackberry Beet Juice

Ingredients:

- 2 beets
- 2 red apples
- 1 cup of blackberries
- ½ inch of fresh ginger
- ½ lemon

Health Benefits:

Blackberries can help to beat inflammation in the body, and help to reduce or eliminate free radicals in the body. Ginger is also anti-inflammatory which makes this juice very powerful against inflammation. Beets will also help detox, by literally helping to push out the toxins due to the betalains which are a group of phytonutrients to help the liver detoxify.

Berry Juice

Ingredients:

- 1 ½ cups of strawberries
- 1 cup of raspberries
- 1 handful of mint leaves

Heath Benefits:

The berries make this juice a highly effective inflammation fighter. Mint can also help with detox and is very soothing to the digestive system while also very pleasant tasting especially when paired with berries.

Fuji Green Juice

Ingredients:

- 4 large Fuji apples

- 1 inch. Piece of fresh ginger

- 1 lemon

- 1 handful of parsley

- 1 handful of basil

Health Benefits:

The soluble fiber, pectin in the apples helps the body prevent plaque buildup in the blood vessels, while the insoluble fibers will help to move toxins out of the digestive system more quickly. The alkaline properties of the lemon paired with the apple makes this juice a powerhouse choice of detoxification. Basil also helps with detox, and specifically targets the kidneys when it comes to toxin elimination. (7)

Coconut Green Juice

Ingredients:

- 1 cup of young coconut meat
- 1 handful of fresh spinach
- ½ of a banana
- 1 handful of kale

Health Benefits:

Leafy greens such as kale, and spinach help to bind toxins for proper removal, while coconut contains strong antibacterial and antiviral properties to help cleanse your body.

Spice Juice

Ingredients:

- 1 fresh mango
- 1 orange
- 1 handful of fresh cilantro
- ½ small jalapeno pepper (Seeded)

Health Benefits:

The spiciness of this juice, from the jalapeno pepper can help you lose weight, and boost your metabolism. The orange will help to give your immune system a boost while the cilantro will help to clear toxins out of your liver.

Veggie Berry Juice

Ingredients:

- 4 carrots
- 1 green apple
- 1 cup of broccoli
- ½ cup of blueberries
- 1 tomato

Health Benefits:

This juice has a wide variety of health benefits. The carrots can help to balance hormones, while the apple can help to prevent plaque buildup in the body. Broccoli is a cruciferous vegetable, which means it is very beneficial for liver detoxification. The blueberries make this juice anti-inflammatory as well, while the tomato can assist with detox and help protect the body from cancer.

Muscle Soother Juice

Ingredients:

- 3 carrots
- 2 stalks celery
- 1 green apple
- 1 cup of broccoli
- 3 spears of asparagus
- 1 handful of fresh parsley
- 1 Tbsp. of olive oil

Health Benefits:

This juice can be used to help sore and achy muscles. When you pair greens with a healthy fat such as olive oil, they are more easily absorbed in the body. The broccoli will help to flush out toxins from the liver, and the asparagus will help with detox since it contains a high amount of glutathione, which is a powerful antioxidant. Asparagus will also help in fighting against the inflammation and pain from achy muscles. Asparagus and celery can also act as diuretics, which can be helpful for those who suffer with high blood pressure.

Pretty in Pink Juice

Ingredients:

- 2 cups of watermelon
- 1 tomato
- 1 lemon

Health Benefits:

Tomatoes can help to protect the body from cancer, while the watermelon can provide your body with hydration and help to flush out toxins along with the lemon, which will help to alkalinize the body.

Back to Your Roots Juice

Ingredients:

- 2 carrots

- 2 small beets

- Sweet potatoes

Health Benefits:

The root vegetables are especially beneficial for your health, and the sweet potato is no exception. Sweet potatoes aide in liver detox as well as beets.

Clean Your Blood Juice

Ingredients:

- 1 cup of Swiss chard
- 4 carrots
- 3 beets
- 1 handful of kale
- 1 handful of fresh parsley

Health Benefits:

If you are looking for a juice to help cleanse the blood this is the one. Between the leafy greens, and the beets, your blood will be thanking you! Parsley is known to help to detoxify the blood, while leafy greens like Swiss chard and kale can also play a part in detoxifying the blood. Swiss chard is also help to help to lower cholesterol.

Love Your Liver Juice

Ingredients:

- 3 carrots
- 1 apple
- 2 beets
- Handful of beet greens
- 2 stalks of celery
- 1 inch of fresh ginger

Health Benefits:

When it comes to detox, you want to be sure you are giving your liver what it needs in order to do its job of detoxification. Beets are one of the best foods you can juice while trying to flush out your liver. Celery can also be helpful, and ginger ca help to combat any inflammation while also soothing the digestive system.

Kale Smoothie (Blend)

Ingredients:

- 1 handful of kale
- 1 apple
- 1 cup of coconut water
- 1 handful of fresh basil

Health Benefits:

Basil will help to flush out toxins, while the apple will help to prevent any plaque buildup in the body. Coconut water is also extremely hydrating and can help provide you with any lost electrolytes. Remember that hydration is essential during detox.

Cocoa Smoothie (Blend)

Ingredients:

- 1 Tbsp. dark cocoa powder
- 1 cup of coconut milk
- 1 frozen banana
- 1 handful of ice

Health Benefits:

Cocoa is high in magnesium and can be very beneficial for heart health. Coconut is also high in properties to help your body to fight infections while also providing you with energy. Bananas can help to keep you feeling full, and prevent you from overeating.

Fat Burning Detox Smoothie (Blend)

Ingredients:

- 1 scoop of plant based protein
- 1 cup of brewed green tea
- 1 mango
- 1 handful of ice

Health Benefits:

If you are looking for a detox smoothie that will help to provide you with energy, and burn fat at the same time, this is a great option! The green tea can help to boost your metabolism, and burn fat, while the protein can help to keep you full and nourish your body with the protein it needs in order to detox.

Calcium Booster Smoothie (Blend)

Ingredients:

- 1 apple
- ½ cup pineapple
- ½ of a frozen banana
- ½ cup of unsweetened Greek yogurt
- 1 tsp of spirulina

Health Benefits:

If you are in need of a calcium boost, this is the smoothie to grab. The Greek yogurt is not only high in protein to keep you full and help stimulate detox, it is also high in calcium. The spirulina is excellent for detox, and is also high in iron.

Congestion Fighting Detox Smoothie (Blend)

Ingredients:

- 2 apples

- 1 lemon

- ½ in of fresh ginger

- Handful of ice

Health Benefits:

Not only is ginger great for fighting inflammation, it can help to clear up congestion which can help to boost detox. The less congestion there is the easier detox is. Lemon is also very cleansing and can help to flush out excess waste as well.

Heart Health Detox Smoothie

Ingredients:

- 2 green apples
- ¼ cup of alfalfa sprouts
- ½ of watercress
- 2 stalks celery
- 2 tsp. wheatgrass powder
- Handful of ice

Health Benefits:

Wheat grass is a powerhouse food that will give your body everything it needs to detox. It is also very alkalinizing and can help to return your body to a more alkaline state. All of the greens in this smoothie are also very healthy for your heart, and can help prevent plaque from clogging vessels while also naturally helping to reduce blood pressure.

Green Grape Juice

Ingredients:

- 1 handful of kale
- 1 cup of green grapes
- 1 cucumber
- 1 granny smith apple

Health Benefits:

Grapes can help to cleanse the body and aide in weight loss. Kale can also help to boost your body's natural detoxing ability while supporting brain and bone health. The cucumber, and apple will also help with removing built up toxins from the body and flush them out through the kidneys.

Immunity Detox Juice

Ingredients:

- 2 apples
- 1 pear
- 1 cup of cherries
- 2 celery stalks

Health Benefits:

This juice is loaded with vitamins to help detox the body and boost the immune system. This juice is especially high in vitamins A and C, which can help build strong bones, and promote skin health.

Antioxidant Powerhouse Juice

Ingredients:

- 1 cup of blueberries

- 1 cup of strawberries

- 1 cup of blackberries

Health Benefits:

All of these berries are loaded with antioxidants, which are going to help to supply your body with what it needs to combat free radicals that are causing inflammation in the body.

Thank you so much for purchasing. I hope it added some value to your life.

Resources

http://life.gaiam.com/article/10-ways-detoxify-your-body

http://www.mindbodygreen.com/0-8404/top-10-reasons-to-detox-when-you-do-it-right.html

http://drhyman.com/blog/2014/03/08/5-reasons-need-detox-5-ways-detox-lose-weight-feel-great/

http://www.bengreenfieldfitness.com/2013/07/how-to-fix-your-gut/

http://www.doctoroz.com/article/3-day-jumpstart-cleanse

http://www.mindbodygreen.com/0-8404/top-10-reasons-to-detox-when-you-do-it-right.html

http://life.gaiam.com/article/10-ways-detoxify-your-body

http://simplegreensmoothies.com/detox-with-herbs

www.ingramcontent.com/pod-product-compliance
Lightning Source LLC
Chambersburg PA
CBHW071125280526
45787CB00003B/1165